The Health Benefits of Black Seed

Mediterranean Miracle Seed

Dr. CASS INGRAM

Knowledge House Publishers

Printed in the United States of America

Disclaimer: This book is not intended as a substitute for medical diagnosis or treatment. Anyone who has a serious disease should consult a physician before initiating any change in treatment

or before beginning any new treatment.

To order this or additional Knowledge House books

call: (909) 284-5620 or order via the web at: www.purelywild.cassingram.com

Contents

Chapter 1

Introduction

T here is a plant that is a blessed creation for all humankind, while largely neglected by the medical profession. Impossible to produce in a laboratory, it is a certain part of the Creative Wisdom that defies explanation. Humans could take advantage of it, gaining immense and wide-ranging benefits. It serves no other major purpose other than as a powerful natural medicine, even though it is edible and is traditionally used in food. This is black seed and its expressed oil.

There is a great deal of confusion regarding this. What is this seed? Is it black cumin? What about black caraway? There is also black sesame. Is it a relative? It has nothing to do with these seeds or the plants from which they are derived. Rather, it is of its own species, notably Nigella sativa. This genus and species is represented by the flowering plants of the buttercup family. Therefore, it is an herbal medicine more than it is a food.

The seeds are particularly strong to taste. Virtually no one will sit and eat a teaspoonful of black seeds. They are too acrid and bitter. A person would only do so for its drug-like effects and only temporarily. As a natural medicine the cold-pressed oil is most palatable and popular, as well as the ground seeds in capsules. Yet, for some people even the oil is objectionable. Thus, there is the option of oil in capsules.

The seed is one of those rare plant components that is actually black in color. The expressed oil has a dark golden color. Most people know of black seed as a nutritional supplement, which they take for specific health complaints or overall wellness. The main supplement available is the pure cold-pressed oil. As well, a person can buy the actual seeds. Yet, few people will use it.

The plant is a shrub of only 18 inches or so tall that grows profusely in hotter climates. Areas where it flourishes include Sudan, Egypt, Ethiopia, Saudi Arabia, India, Pakistan, and Turkey. The heat of the sun has much to do with its aggressive properties. It is generally agreed that the finest oil arises from Turkey, although other respectable sources include Ethiopia and Egypt. The soil in these regions appears to create the richest biochemical profile.

The research on black seed is astounding. This plethora of data proves that it has immense drug-like powers but without the side effects seen in pharmaceuticals. This medicinal capacity has been known since antiquity. Black seed was found in Pharaoh's tomb, apparently both the seed and the oil. The Prophet Muhammad, a spice trader, revived major interest in it when he

said that the seed cured all diseases "except death itself." While the Qur'an doesn't specifically mention it, the spice is described extensively in the Bible. During Islam's height it was heavily prescribed by physicians throughout the Empire. However, in Medieval Europe it seems to be unknown, while in Indian medicine it finds a major place in Ayurvedic practice. Most of this derives from the Prophet's dictate, which served as the stimulus.

In Africa it was routinely popular, as it is today. Africans have a long tradition for the medicinal use of black seed and its oil. Even today, it is held as a universal remedy, typically along with honey, for respiratory complaints.

The real breakthrough is via the findings of modern science. Here, a plethora of properties have been determined that account for its use and popularity. In order to take full advantage of this wondrous medicine for both prevention and cure, let's explore these findings.

Chapter 2

Chemistry and Properties

B lack seed is black. What does this mean in terms of its powers? The seed ripens in a pod and turns this color. There must be much significant capacities in the chemistry that accounts for this. The blackness would imply it is rich in antioxidants and also a vigorous aid for the reddish-black arterial blood. Plus, consider the shape. It looks precisely like a miniature heart, complete with coronary arteries. Look closely with a magnifying glass. It is astounding, glory to God, He sure has a sense of humor. In fact, cardiac issues are the greatest arena for its health benefits. Virtually all heart and circulatory disorders respond to its immense potency.

The chemistry of black seed is telling. It contains potent naturally occurring substances that have a profound impact on health. These substances are the alkaloids, ubiquinones, and phenolic compounds. It is rich in yet other categories, including pigments, melanin being the densest, and sterols, plus hormones. In a testimony to its sophistication some 3% of its total mass remains unidentifiable. Plus, new substances are being found that do not exist in any other plant.

The main active ingredient is a highly metabolically active ubiquinone, known as thymoquinone. This may amount to as high as one percent of the total weight, which is considerable. The typical range is between .7% and 1.2%, which is more than sufficient. In other words, if it is a natural, whole food extract as long as it is within this range the level doesn't matter. There is no use getting caught up in the mechanics of this and falling prey to presumed thymoquinone wars. This is because some purveyors are attempting to gain a market advantage by manipulating the end-product, even adding synthetics. This commonly happens with nutraceuticals, and it is a waste of time and potential. As long as it is truly cold-pressed and from a subtropical Mediterranean region—for instance, Turkey, Egypt, or Ethiopia—that is all that matters.

Coenzyme Q-10 is a similar substance and represents the body's own internally produced ubiquinone. This is an essential nutrient for the metabolism of energy reactions and also oxygen. A person must have sufficient stores to burn this gaseous compound within the cells. To demonstrate how crucial this is if coenzyme Q-10 levels drop within the body by 50% or more, death precipitously ensues. Black seed oil is the richest known source of the vegetable equivalent to this coenzyme. Here, it acts as a replacement for the coenzyme, which is difficult to procure except via synthetics. Thus, since it is virtually impossible to get it in the diet this is the supremely convenient source which anyone can procure. Besides heart tissue top sources include onions, garlic, and shallots. A meal of organic beef or lamb's heart and chopped garlic plus sliced onions would do much to help maintain cardiovascular function. This must be well-chewed, as a person could choke on it. This is because of the elastic, thick connective tissue found in the membrane. The fact is it is just easier to take the black seed oil and/or consume the seeds.

There is so much more to this novel natural medicine than cardiovascular support, though this is considerable. Related to its blackness it is a top source of the pigment melanin, the same one that gives color to darker skin. Black seed contains a number of alkaloids, including types that it alone possesses in goodly quantities such as alpha-heredin. There are also phenolic compounds such as carvacrol, thymol, and carvone. The sterols it contains must be given due consideration. Full of energy these compounds are critical for the strengthening and maintenance of cell membranes, including those of the heart, skin, liver, kidneys, and brain. As well, sterols make the skin smooth and flexible, as they are important for preventing fluid loss from this tissue. They also keep the arteries from degenerating. Simultaneously, sterols help modulate abnormal cholesterol and triglyceride levels. Think of them as God's gift to smoothen all tissues, like the arterial walls, skin tissues, heart muscle, the ducts of the endocrine glands, and mucous membranes.

Chapter 3

Ancient Lore, Compelling Research

The data is in. Black seed and its oil have medicinal properties that are readily proven. The versatility is incredible. A special African journal has outlined this, deeming it effective for nearly a dozen major diseases. This includes disease/syndromes such as asthma, cancer, heart disease, kidney disorders, liver ailments, prostate disorders, breast conditions, and skin diseases. Herbal medicines that have such a versatility of power are few. Thus, black seed and its expressed oil are universal in their scope and may be regarded therapeutic for virtually any condition. The Islamic Prophet in his wisdom said the same, attempting in every way to help people from becoming ill by specifically recommending black seed as a cure.

Both the seed and oil are highly therapeutic. This is true of virtually all manner of syndromes and diseases. Consider the assessment of investigators publishing in the African Journal of Traditional, Complimentary, and Alternative Medicine. It is notable about what they speak. In northern Africa physicians of the Pharaoh's court dispensed black seed for a plethora of conditions, including headaches, colds, bronchial disorders, infections, toothaches, joint disorders, digestive complaints, and allergies. In many ways they were shrewder and more intelligent than the physicians of today because they knew precisely which natural medicines were effective and what to use them for. Pharaoh also discovered that it was invaluable for topical use, including increasing his wives' beauty but also for venomous bites and skin diseases. Much later, Hippocrates, utilized it to reverse liver conditions and digestive disorders, while Dioscorides of the 2nd century found it invaluable to purge worms.

Even so, it wasn't the ancient Egyptians or Greeks who popularized it. If left to them, this would have never happened, and thus it would have been lost into oblivion. It was up to the Prophet Muhammed, may God's peace and blessings be upon him, who in the 7th century did so. In his wisdom and insight, he deemed black seed a universal remedy at a time when no one considered it. He also recommended raw honey and often used the two together. Specifically, he proclaimed, "Make use of black seed (because) it is a cure for every disease: except death." That is a correct revelation made some 1400 years ago, since this is one of the most powerful natural medicines available against heart disease, diabetes, and cancer, the three major killers.

Let us look at the modern research to see if it gives substance to these words. One group of authors insist on major clinical trials, since its actions are "sufficiently understood..." In other words, everyone knows it works. This is to the degree, they comment, that a "drug" could be developed. In other works, since it is so highly effective why not create a monopoly? In contrast, the Prophet's approach was simply to help people, no charge. The authors, writing in the Journal of Pharmacopuncture, stated that there can be no doubt about its actions to reduce blood sugar, excessive blood fats, and as a bronchodilator. It is an impressive assessment about its thoroughness as a medicine. It outlines, along with other investigations, how black seed oil has been shown to act as follows:

•a blood pressure lowering agent

•to fight asthma by loosening secretions and as a bronchodilator

•as a blood sugar-lowering agent

•to reduce blood fat levels and modulate them

•to improve symptoms in chemical warfare victims

•to reduce body weight in obese persons by increasing metabolic rate

•to reduce viral load in hepatitis infections

•to reduce liver toxicity from drug therapy

•to reduce seizure frequency in epilepsy victims

•to improve brain wave function and mental capacities plus attention

•to enhance quality and quantity of sperm

•to cause a higher amount of breast milk production

•to destroy or assist the destruction in H. pylori, ideally with wild oregano oil

•to reduce pain in arthritis, including the rheumatoid type

•to reduce heartburn and stomach pain

This is an immense number of actions for a single natural substance, unheard of in the drug kingdom. Clearly, the intelligence for what the human body needs is found rather than in a laboratory in the domain of almighty God. As the infinitely wise creator He automatically knows what is best for this human race.

Just consider what it does for blood lipids. While reducing the triglycerides and LDL cholesterol it also raises HDL cholesterol levels, an impressive feat. However, that is not all. Black seed oil was found in a mere teaspoon per day to lower hemoglobin A1C, the major marker for early diabetes, while also dropping blood glucose. Clearly, for it to offer such a plethora of functions it is working directly on liver function. In a further investigation the seeds were evaluated, and it was found that in healthy volunteers it led to a significant rise in the white blood cell count. Likewise, the function of the red blood cells was benefited, as measured by a rise in the hemoglobin levels. Both the oil and the seeds have this latter effect. Overall, the oil acts more powerfully than the seeds alone for normalizing blood fat levels. In addition, insulin, that key marker for syndrome X, is reduced—so the combination of this decline plus a lowered hemoglobin A1C act as proof of its antidiabetic actions.

Then, it is no surprise that black seed oil improves brain function, as this organ is the primary consumer of blood sugar in the body. Akhondian and his group demonstrated an anti-seizure capacity for the oil, which is likely related to this phenomenon. Other investigators have determined that it is an antagonist to mental decline and keeps the mind sharp despite aging. This result seems to be related to daily use versus occasional intake.

Pharmaceutical houses take notice

A plethora of scientists and pharmaceutical institutions are attempting to capitalize on black seed. This is through seeking to turn it into a drug. To do so they are attempting to isolate the active ingredients with the scheme of synthesizing them or making single molecule-based medicines. There is another plot to surround the active components with nanotech metals, a completely corrupt process. Yet, black seed contains over 50 active ingredients. Surely, the complex combination of these components are superior to the manipulated or synthetic forms. In fact, there is no way humans can synthesize it, let alone improve upon it by altering its ingredients. In his analysis of its properties E.Z. Dajani and his group called it a substance with "very broad pharmaceutical actions." No wonder the drug companies are attempting to patent it, that is its active ingredients. The reason pharmaceutical companies are doing all in their power to monopolize it can be readily explained. Dajani lists the following actions:

- that it is an antioxidant
- that it is immune modulating
- that it protects cells from aging and toxic destruction
- that it regenerates human cells, including nerve, cardiac, pancreatic, and skin cells
- that it blocks inflammation

Enamored by this, the attempt by pharmaceutical associates to isolate or synthesize the main active ingredient, thymoquinone, has certainly been attempted. Yet, it will not be successful. There is no way an isolated ingredient or synthetic derivative could match the exceedingly immense and sophisticated powers of the original cold-pressed oil.

Those who dismiss natural medicines are confused. Black seed has so many actions and properties that feeble human beings cannot even comprehend it. Just failing to give God credit and understanding the degree of His profound wisdom is more than sufficient reason for their confusion. Let us put it simply. Internally, black seed oil works on five main systems. This is the heart and circulatory tree, the brain, the lungs, the digestive tract, and the kidneys. Who wouldn't benefit from its actions in this regard, as virtually everyone has a disturbance in at least one of these arenas? Plus, it is active for skin health and the vital appearance of the hair as well as nails. There is an element of benefit from this profound herbal medicine for all people. Can this be said about a single drug or even entire categories of them?

Chapter 4

The Nutritious Seed

As far as the typical food-based seeds, such as sunflower, pumpkin, and sesame seeds, as good as they are, none can match the nutritional profile of Nigella sativa. Plus, it is unique in the fact that it contains herbal bitters that act as strong medicines. Bitters, in particular, help stimulate and regulate digestion. Much of the aromatic element is from volatile oils, which account for up to 1.5% of the weight. This oil is what gives it a pungent taste. The seeds are also some 38% fixed or heavy oil, that is monounsaturated and saturated types, along with sterols and other lipids. As well, nigella seed contains albumen, organic acids, flavonoids, and the glucosides, melanthin and metarbin.

As has been stated earlier this is one of those rare natural complexes where a considerable portion consists of substances unknown. This is also true, for instance, of royal jelly. Science cannot fully fathom all its powers either.

As a food seed nigella is nutritionally dense. For instance, it is a good source of calcium, which accounts for some 1% of its total weight. It has nearly an equal density of magnesium, with a tablespoon containing five percent of the daily requirement. Iron, copper, zinc, and manganese are also found in a high density. In one hundred grams or two tablespoonfuls the following mineral density is found:

- 90% of the minimal requirement for copper
- 40% of the daily requirement for zinc
- 22% of the daily need for iron
- 20% of the daily requirement for manganese

Nigella seed is also high in protein, which amounts to an incredible 20% of its weight. The type of protein found in the seeds is highly digestible as well as tissue-building. Impressively, it contains eight of the nine essential amino acids, including rather crucial ones such as tryptophan, phenylalanine, and tyrosine. Both tryptophan and phenylalanine help modulate pain and inflammation and may explain black seed's power in this area. Moreover, tyrosine is critical, as it is needed, in particular, for optimal function of the thyroid gland, which may explain the clinical finding of the boosting for thyroid function. Regardless, its amino acid profile is impressive, which means that it is both a food and medicine and that, as well, whenever possible, it should be added to food and recipes.

Such nutritional density was no surprise to earlier civilizations. It was the Bible which made it clear that the plant was to be raised for its seed, where it was harvested and thrashed with sticks to collect from the fields. Clearly, the people were being instructed or, rather, divinely-inspired to make use of it. Perhaps, this had much to do with the rather low rate of degenerative disease, including heart disorders, in that era. The 11th century Islamic physician al- Biruni described it as a harvested crop, calling it a grain.

Recently, it was discovered that black seed is a dense source of the rather rare pigment melanin. This is the same substance that gives human skin darker color as seen in Asians, Middle Easterners, and Africans. Found in the outer coatings of the seeds this pigment is one of the most powerful natural medicines known and is, in particular, a potent antioxidant. This makes sense, since within the skin it has the capacity to protect cells against the harshness of ultraviolet radiation. Melanin also has hormone-like powers. The high density of this pigment may explain its historical use by the ancient Egyptians for skin health.

There are a plethora of saponins in nigella seeds, the primary one being the glycoside and pigment alpha-hederin, also known as melanthin. Nigella seed also contains alkaloids, notably indazole and nigelicine as well as the novel nigellimine. Other active ingredients include the alkaloid nigellidine. This compound contains a special chemical center, known as an indazole nucleus, one of only two known. In fact, continuously, new, never-before-known compounds are being discovered in black seed.

Nigella seed is a good source of vitamin E, containing various analogues, including alpha, beta, and gamma. As well, the so-called unsaponifiable component of black seed contains unique lipids. These lipids have never been isolated from any oilseed and include dienoate and monoesters. In addition, goodly amounts of beta sitosterol, campesterol, and stigmasterol are found in the fixed oil fraction. Of such sterols beta sitosterol accounts for some 70% of the content. This sterol is well known for its biological activity in supporting heart health and for the integrity of cell membranes. All such plant sterols are exceptionally heart- healthy. There is even an FDA-allowed claim for them.

The discovery of certain of these components confirms the novel nature of black seed compared to all other oilseeds. For instance, as has been alluded to within the seed mass six rare indazole-class alkaloids have been recently discovered, including two that were previously unknown, a methylnigelidine component and the compound, nigelanoid. These compounds are pigments and thus are similar in their actions to melanin. The point is this is a finely created complex. No human can imitate it. In the attempt to do so they will corrupt it.

The vitamin content of black seeds is impressive. It is the seeds which are the richest source. The following are what is found in 100 grams or about two tablespoons:

- •80% of the daily need for thiamine
- •35% of the daily requirement for niacin
- •10% of the daily requirement for folic acid
- •35% of the minimum needs for vitamin B6
- •5% of the daily requirement for riboflavin

.

This is an extremely high amount for so little of weight. Few other food substances offer such a density of these metabolically critical catalysts. Both niacin and thiamine are crucial for energy metabolism and are required for the efficient burning of carbohydrates. In particular, niacin is required for hormone synthesis. As well, both these vitamins are crucial for the production of brain chemicals known as neurotransmitters, including the anti-depressant substance tryptophan. Essentially, the combustion of all fuel sources within the cells, particularly, the burning of glucose is dependent upon both niacin and thiamine. Both of these metabolic giants are required for the efficient function of that intracellular energy producing mechanism, known as the Kreb's Cycle.

However, the most important chemical constituents, which account for its medicinal powers, are the aromatic compounds, thymoquinone, thymol, carvone, and carvacrol. Of these, thymoquinone is the most crucial.

Yet, is thymoquinone itself a nutrient? It can surely be said to be so, since it acts much coenzyme Q-10, which is vitamin-like.

Thymoquinone to the rescue

The primary active ingredient of black seed is thymoquinone. An essential oil it is related to the phenolic compound thymol, though a unique, edible form of this molecule. Thymoquinone can be removed or isolated for use as a drug. However, for therapeutic purposes it is best to leave it in its naturally occurring configuration in the seed or oil. A benzoquinone, it is a phenolic compound with immense medicinal actions. Versus thymol, it possesses additional oxygen molecules complexed to a benzene ring, the latter containing double bonds. Thymoquinone has a diversity of powers, and Nigella sativa seed is the densest source in all nature. Other rich sources include plants of the bergamot species, such as Citrus aurantium, a type of inedible bitter orange, and purple bergamot, which is also known as bee balm. Another good source is juniper. Thus, truly, thymoquinone is rare to the extreme. In fact, black seed and juniper represent the only major source readily

available. Of note, a black seed oil-juniper essential oil supplement is available. in raw honey it is ultra- potent for supporting overall health, especially of the respiratory and renal systems. It is also an agent to flush heavy metals from the system.

One of the main mechanisms of action of this compound relates to its antioxidant powers. Thymoquinone has the capacity to quench noxious free radicals in a dominating way. In fact, this is with the same force as the all-important enzyme-based antioxidant, superoxide dismutase. Another key mechanism of action relates to its anti-inflammatory powers. This is also a consequence of its antioxidant actions, as thymoquinone blocks lipid peroxidation in cell membranes, the latter being a major cause of tissue inflammatory reactions.

Chapter 5

How To and How Much

B lack seed works best if it is a regular part of the dietary and supplement regimen. It is difficult to take too much. Rather, the typical approach is to consume too little. Truly, the key is daily use. This is how it offers the greatest protection against tissue degeneration. There is much desire to know the dosage, how much is too little and what amount is too much. The first issue that must be clarified is that it is non-toxic. Generally, if using a high-quality source of truly cold-pressed oil, there isn't a too much situation. No one is going to take it foolishly. Top quality, truly cold-pressed black seed can be taken with impunity. Commentary about toxicity, largely found on the Internet, is bogus. The fact is in certain disease processes the only way to rectify them is through large doses. This is especially true of heart, lung, and skin disorders as well as cancer.

Types of products

There are a number of black seed supplements which offer unique formulas and the highest quality. Let us review the list to understand their nature, best sources of quality, and the benefits that people can derive. Emphasis will be on combination supplements, where the black seed is synergized by the added ingredients.

Black seed oil, straight

It doesn't really matter, but some people prefer black seed oil straight with nothing added. Yet, though it might be little known, readily, black seed and its oil gain an additive effect by certain formulations. Even so, for instance, the spice oils which are added to it may account for a small percentage per bottle or capsule, like 2% to 5% for example. The consumer is getting even more value than in the 100% oil by getting additional spice nutrients. Even so, pure cold-pressed black seed oil is available typically in an eight- ounce container. It can be consumed in a dosage of a tsp. or two daily. It may also be taken every other day. Yet, the point is to gain the benefits it should be taken regularly.

Black seed oil with added spice oils

There is a value to added Mediterranean-source spice oils. These act as antioxidants, keeping the oil fresh, plus act as penetrating agents. The spice oils facilitate the absorption and utilization of the black seed oil. This is the ideal type for applying to the skin, as it contains oils of rosemary and oregano. There are a few such black seed oil supplements on the market.

Cardiac-supporting pomegranate- and muscadine-infused oil

Black seed oil has a strong taste. To have a flavored oil is a major benefit. Yet, these are not mere flavorings. Mediterranean pomegranate concentrate adds yet another layer of protection, specifically for the cardiovascular system. Dense in punicalagins it offers a major additive benefit by impacting the health of the arterial tree but also the heart muscle itself. There is yet another aspect, which is its rich supply of ellagic acid. The supplement also contains muscadine skin extract, a dense source of resveratrol. Imagine having thymoquinone, alpha-heredin, ellagic acid, punicalagins, punic acid, and resveratrol all in one: nothing can overcome it.

As well, it has the divine code behind it. This combines the best of all Qur'anic and biblical medicines: black seed, grape, and pomegranate. God knows what He is doing, and by mentioning these specifically this is attempted guidance for humankind, while virtually no one pays heed to it.

Mediterranean pomegranate concentrate is of the highest quality known. The punic acid component, found mainly in the seeds, is similar to conjugated linoleic acid, the substance in grass-fed meat that is heart healthy. The various flavonoids, like ellagic acid, exhibit high antioxidant activity, preventing age- related oxidative damage to the heart and arteries.

This might seem simple and not high-tech enough, but it is true. After all, it is just grapes, pomegranate, and a spicy-tasting seed. How could they do anything beyond the powers of modern medicine? In fact, indisputably, these foods are more powerful in aiding the body than any synthetic drug. Consider again the chemistry. In black seed oil there is thymoquinone, the coenzyme Q-10-like molecule, while pomegranate provides ellagic acid and the muscadine, resveratrol. Back seed oil offers alpha-heredin, nigellone, melatonin, and plant sterols plus a high density of vitamins and minerals, while pomegranate is dense in potent flavonoids as well as vitamin C. Together, there is immense synergy in this combination. In fact, such a complex is an authoritative remedy for all that might afflict the heart and circulatory tree. These are oxygenating complexes, agents that increase arterial elasticity, substances which block clotting, and agents which decrease excess lipids. For reasons humans cannot fathom almighty God favors them all and mentions them specifically in His holy books, saying they will be among the fruit of paradise. Perhaps, if this became popularized from an early age, this three-in-one complex, there would be no heart disease. It is certainly superior to succumbing to all manner of invasive treatment, as is demonstrated by the following case history:

CASE HISTORY:

Mr. N. is a 60-year-old man who for a variety of reasons suffered a multiplicity of cardiac issues that left him with 18 stints. As a result, he suffered continuous failure of heart function and hypertension. After taking the black seed oil pomegranate-muscadine combination he some 5 T. daily, his blood pressure quickly normalized, and all his cardiac symptoms were minimized. To keep himself heart healthy he takes this cardiac-supporting triple formula daily.

Raw honey- and wild juniper-infused oil

This is based on an ancient remedy of combining black seed oil with raw, wild honey, two of the Creative Mind's finest. Humans must always keep in mind that they did not make these natural medicines. Plus, in a million years they could never synthesize anything remotely similar. Attempting to exceed His magnificent powers is a useless endeavor. Always, the end product is compromised. These natural medicines are gifts, and they must be appreciated in this way. God is so powerful that He creates them in a flash, and there is no way the human can understand this. Optimally, we can also mix the powers of wild oregano oil with wild high-mountain juniper oil.

This is a simple combination but one that cannot be matched in potency, specifically for respiratory, cardiac, digestive, and renal complaints. Once again, the complexes show real power—that power and potency of synergy and positive interactions—over the plain oil alone. Juniper is an immense aid to the entire respiratory system as well as the kidneys, where it acts as a cleansing agent—but so does the oregano, black seed, and honey. Of note, like black seed, juniper is one of those rare sources of thymoquinone. Thus,

the two together are the ultimate powerhouse. The kind creator made these medicines for us. There is only benefit, often profoundly so, from taking them, as demonstrated by the following:

CASE HISTORY:

Ms. P. had a history of a bizarre condition where she became extremely congested at night, mainly in her sinus region. Her whole face felt stuffed up, and she couldn't do anything about it. Taking raw honey with black seed oil and juniper oil, she consumed two dropperfuls at night. Dramatically, all her congestion symptoms were eliminated. She continues to take the formula at a lesser dose, always at night to gain the benefit.

Black seed with organic yacon

Because of black seed oils rather strong, acrid taste it is ideal to have formulas which have an improved taste profile. This is one of the benefits of the oil added into an organic yacon syrup base. Both the oil and the yacon are raw, which is a special benefit. Such a formula offers the added effect of being a probiotic. Plus, both black seed and yacon are involved with normalization of metabolism plus weight control. This would be an ideal formula for the stimulation of healthy weight loss. It is also optimal for children and the elderly, who might resist the taste profile. Plus, it makes an optimal addition to smoothies and possibly desserts, which it gives an inviting picante taste.

Black seed

The seeds of the plant themselves are a medicinal complex. A person just has to find a way to consume them. About a half teaspoon or full teaspoon per day is therapeutic. Chewed on, their therapeutic power hits the body hard and strong. If cooked, the power is less. It is the raw seed that should be taken advantage of. The seeds can be sprinkled on a salad or at the end of cooking of soup. In stir fry it gives added taste, once again towards the end of cooking. They may even be added to smoothies. Research shows that the raw seeds have immense immune potentiating properties; the intake increases both the activity and count of white blood cells. All people could benefit from this. Even a greater potentiation would be achieved when combined with wild oregano therapy.

Black seeds have major metabolic actions on metabolism. They speed the burning of cellular fuel, thus preventing fat deposition. The seeds also help block the excessive risk in sugar levels from carbohydrate meals. As far as the digestion the raw seeds, well chewed, acts as a digestive stimulant as well as a potent antiparasitic agent. For those who can't handle the taste or lack the discipline the pulverized seeds in a capsule are an option.

Black seed capsules of ground seed plus red sour grape and brown cumin seed

If possible, ground black seed should also be mixed with added brown cumin and red sour grape, which are synergistic to its profile. In overall therapeutic powers this is superior to the seeds alone. This formula is an ideal therapeutic to take with the oil of black seed. It makes a most delicious addition to various foods, including cream cheese, cottage cheese, yogurt, soup, and stir fry.

Black seed oil with fennel and cumin seed oils

This is a spectacular combination of what amounts to the maximum synergy in a black seed capsule. As always, the oil should amount to 95% or more of the content, with the other medicinal agents added as potent synergists. Cumin oil works strongly with the black seed oil in blood sugar control, acting as an insulin-like agent. Fennel is a stimulant for liver function, notably the synthesis and outpouring of bile. Healthy for the pancreas it is also a specific remedy for hookworm. Cumin is yet another worm-killer and is aggressive against the eggs, as is oregano oil. That means there are four worm-purging agents in this complex, making the formula highly medicinal. Regarding rosemary, this is one of the most potent fat-soluble antioxidants known. The fatty tissues of the body, notably the brain and spinal cord, are greatly protected by its routine use. Once it enters the brain and spinal cord it prevents age-related degeneration of these organs. It also blocks the aging process of all cells in the body by acting on the cell membranes. Oregano oil is included because it, too, is a stimulating substance. An antioxidant, it works in a different way than rosemary. Wild oregano oil is a water-phase antioxidant, that is it has its guarding action in the fluids within the body.

Chapter 6

Beauty, Inside and Out

With all its profound utility for the internal system it is easy to lose track of its beautifying effects. Black seed oil can make a person both feel and look extra beautiful. It does this to the skin, face, hair, and nails. Oil of black seed was one of the secrets for the extraordinary beauty of Queen Nefertiti, who was admired for her exquisite complexion. An avid user Nefertiti made use of black seed oil by applying it on her face and hair. Notes D. A. S. Hussein in her investigative report published in *NetJournals,* the Queen also used it to give luster to her nails, that is she soaked her nails. Cleopatra also relied upon it, apparently applying it to her face and hair. These elegant ones knew it kept their skin smooth and beautiful despite the harsh climate and the onset of aging.

Today, it can be used in the same way. The best oil for this purpose contains small amounts of wild rosemary and oregano oils. Simply gently rub or apply on the face at night. Also take it internally, at least a teaspoonful daily. By doing so it dramatic changes may occur, as demonstrated by the following:

CASE HISTORY:

Ms. U. is a 60-year-old female concerned about aging impact on her facial skin. As a result, she opted for the Nefertiti treatment of applying black seed oil on her face. The treatment was done regularly every night. After 30 days she experienced an astonishing result. Literally, her face peeled off, that is she had a shedding of her epithelial layer. This was not dissimilar to a snake that sheds its coat. The result was astonishing. She looked fully 20 years younger.

Obviously, the oil is highly sophisticated in its actions upon human skin cells. Imagine the good it does on the inside of the body. So, it can always be utilized in both ways. The various topical formulas available include:

•A pure oil with added wild rosemary and oregano oils

•A 5% to 10% black seed oil emollient cream with Canadian balsam, raw honey, and bee propolis

•the black seed oil 5% shampoo and conditioner free of all chemical additives

•the black seed oil dental pull for oral detoxification with oils of clove bud and wild oregano

In all cases the health of the hair, skin, and nails is greatly aided by internal consumption. What a benefit it is that it can be utilized in both ways. In all cases of chronic skin diseases, the internal intake of the oil is a mainstay. Perhaps the best one is the cold- pressed oil with wild rosemary and oregano oils. Then, if the cream is added, this would produce stupendous results. The same is true of the simultaneous use of the shampoo and conditioner. With the latter a modest amount should be left in the hair after rinsing. Plus, the oil can be

relied on as a nail soak for diseases of that system or for strengthening
them.

Chapter 7

Diseases and Syndromes

There are countless illnesses and syndromes which respond significantly to black seed's therapeutic powers. This "blessed seed" and its extracts thus must be a front-line medicinal substance for disease processes, including a number of significant ones. The general value in various conditions has been alluded to. Let's look at the specifics:

Heart disease

This is black seed oil's greatest arena for potency. Definitely God's gift for this organ system, it has been already stated that the seed is heart-shaped, a novel finding discovered here. That means a great deal, since in this book homage is given to almighty God and His forces for such an astounding creation. Regardless, how did He do this? It is a mystery. Thus, this heart look-alike can be no coincidence. It is as if to say, "Alright, you humans, let us see if you are smart enough to figure this out."

It is this substance which has direct actions on the heart muscle, while also doing the astounding and unexpected. It has the capacity to work directly on the central mechanism: the cardiac centers within the brain stem. Even so, black seed works on the heart and circulation in a number of ways. The thymoquinone aids in oxygen metabolism within the heart cells and also the arterial walls. Black seed contains a multitude of components that have positive actions on blood fats, as follows:

•reduction of triglyceride content

•reduction of LDL cholesterol.

•increase in HDL cholesterol levels

•when combined with cumin and fennel lowering of total cholesterol

Pulverized black seed also has specialized actions on the heart, especially if combined with that other godly remedy, Mediterranean-source low-sugar, dried red sour grape. This combination is supremely potent for regulating blood fat levels and also enhancing arterial health.

Hypertension

There are as many as 60,000 miles of blood vessels in the human arterial and venous systems, and they need all the help they can have. One of these helping aids is thymoquinone- and nigellone-rich black seed oil. Here, it should be kept in mind that the oil and seed are muscle relaxants, and they are capable specifically of causing relaxation or normalization of tension in the arterial walls. The disease is directly related to excess stress and tension.

Virtually no case of hypertension can resist the curative powers of black seed. Of all herbal medicines it is authoritative for this condition. In many instances nothing but this is needed, especially if taken as a combination with pomegranate and muscadine. People often make this too complicated, as do nutritional companies. It is not necessary to consume an excess of supplements, massive amounts of vitamins, esoteric herbs, and mega-doses of minerals to reverse this condition. Grape extracts, pomegranate concentrate, and black seed oil are sufficient, while in stubborn conditions it may be necessary to add the unrefined, crude sour grape powder. The oregano, especially the crude herb with garlic and onion, as well as the aromatic juice, may also prove effective. In addition, the oil may provoke a temporary rise in blood pressure, which can be significant. Over time, this reaction typically dissipates, and the oregano oil may act as an aid in the elimination. In all cases where oregano oil is needed the black seed oil must also be taken. The power of this oil is demonstrated by the following case history:

CASE HISTORY:

Mr. T. is a 60 year-old male with stubborn hypertension. Resistant to the medication, which he had taken for decades, he opted to consume black seed oil. His blood pressure had risen to 230 over 180. There was great concern the person might drop over and die or have a stroke. His son-in-law gave him the black seed oil but in an incredibly high dose: one-fourth cup or more daily. Within a week the blood pressure fell virtually to normal at a level of 140 over 90.

Diabetes

In all cases, whether type 2 or the more uncommon type 1, black seed is a therapy of choice. Both the seed and the oil work directly upon those specialized pancreatic cells, known as beta islet cells, which are responsible for insulin production. The optimal black seed oil supplement also contains cumin, fennel, rosemary, and oregano, all of which act as antidiabetic agents. As well, the pulverized seed with red sour grape and ground cumin is yet another optimal supplement.

The two together may help reverse this condition and will also reduce hemoglobin A1c levels plus blood sugar levels.

Cancer

Black seed has immense value to support the fight against this condition. It has that novel property of stimulating the immune system against any invader. The immune system has a love affair with black seed whenever a person consumes it. It causes an increase in both the count and the activity of white blood cells. Recent studies have shown that the thymoquinone content is responsible for strong anticancer properties. Specifically, it can influence apoptosis, which is programmed cell death. It is particularly active in this regard against leukemia, brain cancer, breast tumors, and intestinal cancers. Yet, for any internal carcinoma black seed is indicated.

Psoriasis/eczema

As a source of omega 3s, 6s, and 9s black seed oil has regenerative actions on the skin. With eczema and psoriasis this is often complicated by infection, notably by parasites and fungi. Black seed kills these. The result is the liberation of skin health because the organ is a barometer of health or lack of it in the gut. In particular, psoriasis is directly related to worm infestation, notably by intestinal and liver flukes. With eczema, typically, the concern is primarily fungus. To act in concert with the black seed oregano juice is suggested as well as the multiple spice oil capsules. These appear to be even more potent for these conditions than oregano oil itself. A black seed oil cream in an emollient base of Canadian balsam plus propolis, is a highly effective and soothing topical treatment. It can be applied repeatedly until the skin disorder/lesion is eliminated, speeded greatly by internal consumption of black seed.

H. pylori

For this disorder black seed oil is a boon. This is particularly true of the capsules containing oils of cumin and fennel, both of which are major substances for digestive support. The primary cause of GERD and esophageal reflex, this is an agent which infects the entire lining of the stomach. If not eliminated, eventually H. pylori causes hypochlorhydria and stomach cancer. Black seed oil aids in the killing of this perpetrator, but it is most effective when combined with wild oregano oil. Together, they will efficiently eradicate this pathogen.

Gallbladder disorders and gallstones

With any type of stone black seed is the answer, especially gallstones. It acts to both dissolve and purge them. Plus, its regular intake is highly preventive against gallstone formation. Generally, people will notice that after a monthly course there is improvement, which may be noticed on ultrasound. Ideal formulas include black seed oil with wild oregano and rosemary oils and capsules with added fennel and cumin oils. A potent dosage is to take a T. twice daily or five capsules twice daily. Another option is the total body purging agent, which is extremely aggressive, and complexes of wild, raw greens with black seed oil. Routinely, this formula thoroughly purges/dissolves stones from this organ.

Hepatitis

In this condition, typically, there is infection within the liver cells by viruses. Even so, another form is known as chemical hepatitis or that resulting from alcohol ingestion. With the viruses there is hepatitis A, B, C, and E along with Epstein-Barr infection. It is irrelevant which one it is, as black seed and its expressed oil are effective for all. At the minimum the oil will continually purge the liver, causing it to make additional bile. Its actions on this condition are greatly enhanced by the oil of oregano as well as the juice-essence. This is a triplicate combination which is exceptionally powerful. The ideal black seed oil for liver support contains the seed oils of fennel and cumin plus wild rosemary oil.

Constipation

In constipation black seeds and their expressed oil find much efficacy. This is largely because of their role as bile stimulants. It also relates to their action on vitalizing liver and intestinal wall function. Plus, parasites are a major cause of this disorder, and black seed obliterates them. There is also a fungal element to this condition, particularly by Candida albicans. Yet, this largely meets its match with the black seed, especially if combined with wild oregano oil.

Hemorrhoids

In the fight against hemorrhoids black seed is essential, both topically and internally. Mix black seed oil cream with raw honey and Canadian balsam and apply as an emollient. Its content of thymoquinone is effective against both the internal and external types. This is a potent anti-inflammatory and analgesic agent, which makes its topical application and internal consumption ideal. Plus, it gets at the root cause of many cases, which is congestion in the intestinal system. This congestion may be caused by worms, which black seed decimates. It may also be a consequence of a sluggish liver, which it activates. Black seed causes a strong production of bile, which greatly aids the digestive process. It also helps eliminate constipation, and this is a major factor in this syndrome.

Kidney disorders

Nigella sativa has shown positive effects in reversing kidney pathology. In fact, it has been shown to induce the development

of new kidney cells in the repair of this organ. In renal failure it may be effective, largely by increasing oxygenation within diseased cells.

In a study by Bayrak and his group it was found to improve serum BUN and creatinine levels. This is a major achievement. If taken with pomegranate and muscadine, there is even greater positive impacts, as both these acidic fruit sources are urinary stimulants. Within the kidney tissue the antioxidant enzymes superoxide dismutase, catalase, and glutathione peroxidase were all increased. Thus, black seed acted to assist kidney cells in scavenging free radicals to prevent inevitable tissue damage. Additionally, thymoquinone has been found to aid in the destruction and purging of kidney stones. If a person is in the midst of such stones, even passing them, black seed oil, especially the type with muscadine and pomegranate, must be consumed. The same is true during the crisis of kidney failure.

Pancreatic disorders

For all pancreatic disorders black seed is essential. Well tolerated, this is even true of pancreatitis and cancer of this organ. This is greatly enhanced when combined with oil of wild oregano, along with its aromatic juice. If all three are taken together, this can have extraordinary effects on the tissues. A person should take these supplements as aggressively as necessary to calm this organ, which may require doses taken several times daily. A typical protocol would be the capsules or oil, about two capsules at a time or a teaspoon of the oil at least four times daily. The oil of oregano, edible type and wild, must be taken at a dose of five to ten drops, again four or more times daily or as capsules, one or

two at a time. The juice can be consumed even more aggressively, an ounce or more four or more times daily. If there is obstructive pancreatic disease, the juice should be the focus. Even an entire bottle per day can be consumed.

Intestinal parasites

Over 5000 years ago black seed was relied upon as a vermifuge, meaning it killed worms or drove them out of the body. Modern research confirms this. In a study by Egyptian investigators, it was found to impede the growth of or kill the pandemic pathogen, Schistosoma mansoni, in all its phases, even the eggs. In destroying these eggs, it worked better than the tested drugs, when it killed them directly along the intestinal walls. In another evaluation it was tested in children against cestode worms. Here, once again, it was found to kill efficiently the noxious agent, far more effective than the standard, chloroquine.

Rabbits were tested which were infested with coccidiosis. The black seed oil especially was able to destroy these germs, resulting in weight gain and revived vigor. The same occurs in human children and adults. Once the parasites are obliterated, which black seed can achieve, failure to thrive, a common consequence, is curtailed. Victims now can put on weight and, if they are anemic, gradually build back their blood. The parasites must be completely purged. This is the only way the individual can thrive. To do so it may be necessary to add other key antiparasitic complexes such as the total body purging agent, the multiple spice oil complex, and the juice or essence of wild oregano.

Vitiligo

Vitiligo is a pigment disorder characterized by an intensive disturbance in the function of certain pigment-producing skin cells, known as melanocytes. Rich in melanin, black seed oil is an ideal therapy. After all, the disease is related to a loss of this pigment from the skin tissues. To treat vitiligo take it internally and apply topically. In one study, 33 vitiligo patients were evaluated. Given a cream containing the oil they were monitored for six months, while it was applied twice daily. Significant reversal of the pigment loss was observed, even on the genitals. It was stated that a black seed oil-based cream is a dependable treatment for vitiligo, especially in sensitive regions such as the genitals. To treat this condition and to induce regeneration of the skin layers apply the black seed oil emollient cream with Canadian balsam, spruce resin, and bee propolis, two to four times daily. Also, take the oil of black seed, one or two tablespoons daily.

Alopecia

In certain dramatic cases black seed oil has caused restitution of lost hair due to alopecia. This is patchy hair loss caused by a fungus, which infects the scalp. The causative agent, a normal flora resident, pityriasis, turns pathogenic for causes unknown, although excessive sugar intake, stress, and hormonal disturbances are key factors. With a 5% black seed oil shampoo and conditioner it can be treated topically. Plus, the oil can be rubbed into the scalp. In addition, it must be consumed internally, at least one T. daily. If it is a tough case, 2 T. can be consumed twice daily.

Male pattern baldness (also, hair loss in females)

Make no mistake black seed oil is a hair-growth agent. This is true both topically and internally. Through the use of a 5% black seed shampoo and conditioner there are visible benefits. Yet, it works best if taken internally. Topically, there is benefit by simply rubbing the scalp-activating oil on the scalp and by regularly using black seed oil-based shampoo, while avoiding all shampoos that contain chemicals and toxins.

Chronic fatigue syndrome

In all cases the intake of black seed and its expressed oil benefit energy production. If a person is tired, such a one will generally not be after taking black seed, for instance, in the morning. For best results consume with oils of cumin, fennel, and rosemary. Cumin and fennel oils create added energy by helping to regulate blood sugar and also stimulating healthy digestion. To accentuate the results also consume wild oregano oil, at least one to two drops twice daily.

Obesity

One of black seed's great claims to fame is its capacities against obesity. This is largely a result of its immense powers of increasing metabolism, known as thermogenesis. Black seed, both the seed component and the oil, is a dependable weight loss aid. The oil is greatly enhanced with the addition of other spice

oils, notably oils of fennel, cumin, and rosemary. As a result of intake, the metabolic rate may rise by as much as 35%, which is highly significant.

The body has no choice. When something this pungent and spicy is ingested, metabolically, it must react. Plus, thymoquinone acts strongly to increase the burning of oxygen in the cells, and that means a greater amount of fuel, glucose and more, will be combusted. Just think of an internal combustion machine that has the right exact octane of fuel to work efficiency. Black seed oil is just that fuel to achieve maximum capacity. To enhance the burning of fat take the black seed oil and multiple spice oil capsules, three or more caps twice daily, along with the oil, one or more tsp. daily.

Regardless, it is possible to determine metabolic oxygen deficiency. This is by looking at the cuticle-area half-moons. If these regions of the proximal nail beds are lacking these half-moons, this is proof of deficiency of cellular oxygen. Through the consumption of black seed oil, especially if mixed with muscadine and pomegranate concentrates, this can readily be reversed. Pay no attention to the pinky and thumb; moons here are irrelevant.

Breast milk production

In traditional medicine Nigella sativa is known as a galactagogue, which means inducer of breast milk. In a rat study this property was evaluated. A black seed extract was found to increase milk production by as much as 37%, an impressive feat for a single herbal medicine. This was thought likely a result of the induction of prolactin, which, regardless, black seed oil contains. Only a few herbs meet this profile. In traditional medicine black seed is well-respected for its ability to induce milk production. In some areas it is routinely given to all new mothers, so their milk stays rich and flowing.

Professor Ali Esmail Al-Snafi has proven this. He found that it had a direct action on pituitary production of this hormone, likely because of an action on the nerves responsible for its release from this gland. Thus, it has an intelligence to cause the brain to 'order' breast milk production. Furthermore, it is completely safe and beneficial for all breast-feeding as well as pregnant women. Even so, in early pregnancy it is best to take it in reasonable amounts, like one teaspoon, then increasing the dose towards the middle of pregnancy.

Infertility

There is an element in black seed that makes it universally special. It is doing all that is listed for the body, and it also acts on the fertility mechanism? In one placebo-controlled human trial it was found to act impressively on men. The consumption of black seed oil caused an increase in sperm count, semen volume, and motility. In females it aids greatly in normalizing the menstrual cycle. It has been also shown to increase progesterone levels, which always aids in fertility. Incredibly, it also appears to increase the counts of vital, active follicles, while also improving the function and structure of the corpus luteum. In both males and female's testosterone levels are increased. This is confirmed by so- called folk use, as infertile couples are often told to consume both the oil and the seed. In a rat study high doses were found to "increase fertility potential" by raising the levels of LH and testosterone, that is both the follicles, and the sperm are more well prepared as a result of its intake.

Menstrual disorders

It is no surprise that black seed is optimal for the menstrual cycle. This complex is rich in hormones that mimic those needed for a woman's cycle. Found within the oil are considerable amounts of key hormonal substances, including estradiol, progesterone, and testosterone. There is even prolactin, which is relatively rare. There is FSH and LH, two key pituitary-based hormones needed for menstrual regulation and fertility. A reasonable amount, like two capsules or a teaspoon daily, could act as a menstrual regulator.

For post-menopausal syndrome there is much value. After all, it is a relatively dense source of estrogenic compounds, but not the type that could cause issues such as tumor growth, uterine fibroids, or cancer. In fact, rather, the ingestion helps reverse these. The findings of a number of studies indicate that because of its natural, raw hormones black seed is an optimal "hormone replacement" complex for post-menopausal women. Its consumption even aided in reversing vaginal dryness, likely a result of its plant estrogen content.

Mental disturbances

The list of mental disorders aided by black seed is impressive. At researchgate.com it is listed as an "excellent nutraceutical for brain function." What is meant by that? It is the fact that consistent use "significantly improves brain function," making it a valid treatment for depression, anxiety, epilepsy, and memory loss. It is also noted that it contains a number of substances, including thymoquinone, which aid in nerve cell repair. In a study by Imam and his group, artificially created amnesia was evaluated. They discovered that the oil for only 14 days halted the drug-induced amnesia syndrome to such a degree that they deemed it a "promising anti-amnesia agent..." and that it must therefore undergo clinical trials.

Chronic pain

There is value in black seed oil for pain and inflammation syndromes. It can be applied topically and is typically effective. Its content of the highly oxygenating compound thymoquinone accounts for its powers internally in blocking the inflammatory response. As well, it can be applied as a 5% emollient cream with wild rosemary oil plus Canadian balsam and bee propolis. For best results rub on and take the oil daily. For extra power take the wild, raw whole food turmeric drops, 10 or more drops twice daily.

Asthma

Besides heart disease another major focus for black seed is respiratory diseases. This is especially true of asthma, where black seed and its oil have been represented by a number of clinical trials. In these evaluations it has been determined that it is more effective than medication, while decreasing the need for inhalant drugs. Further, it has a direct action on the bronchial tract, causing smooth muscle relaxation and therefore decreasing bronchospasm. The specialist formula of the oil with wild juniper and raw honey is particularly effective against this condition. Crude, raw honey also has a specialist action for bronchial and lung health. For best results take oil of black seed and mix with juniper and raw honey.

In these various conditions listed black seed should be expected to produce significant results. The data is behind it. Yet, if further support is needed, it can be combined with wild oregano-based supplements such as the oil. For pain and inflammation syndromes, it may be enhanced by the addition of wild, raw turmeric complex with ginger and rosemary. For psoriasis and eczema, take black seed oil along with wild, raw chaga, is also productive. In the need for kidney support wild, a raw cranberry extract may be a beneficial addition. For brain and neurological function wild, raw turmeric plus raw hemp or cannabis extract could increase the results. It is never one natural medicine alone to allow for optimization. The combination effect is exceedingly powerful. This may be to such a degree that the potency and effectiveness may prove astounding, to lay public and medical professionals alike.

Chapter 8

Conclusion

B lack seed is a great blessing for this entire human race. It influences a plethora of functions offering wide-ranging benefits, acting vigorously on the entire body and all its organs. It can be seen that black seed has a number of novel uses, including the treatment of rather difficult-to-cure, bizarre conditions such as infertility, vitiligo, alopecia, and deficiency in breast milk. Plus, it acts on the common ones, including heart diseases, hypertension, diabetes, arthritis, and intestinal disorders. That makes it one of the most novel natural medicines known, far exceeding the powers of any drug.

The way it must be consumed is in the most unaltered form possible. More important than the content of any single active ingredient is the means by which it is produced and where it grows. The finest black seed arises from the heart of the Middle East such as Turkey. Other decent sources arise from Egypt and Ethiopia, with India-grown being of a lesser quality. It is generally held though, that the seeds from Turkey and the Levant are the highest in quality. They do seem to have the most robust aroma and flavor, and they are more bitter to taste, a good sign. Ideally, oil from this region is the optimal choice.

The other issue is that it must be exclusively cold-pressed. The application of heat or solvents leads to its degradation. This oil is easily damaged by processing. Another element of concern is standardization. It is impossible to do so with the oil without corruption. For instance, there is no such thing as standardized black seeds, cumin seeds, or sesame seeds. While cheaper, standardization is the lowest quality and even suspect in the method of production.

Fortification, though, can be a positive issue. This is through the addition of spice oils which greatly boost the power and efficacy. As well, these substances offer an antioxidant function which prevents the oil from degradation. If it can be procured, the combination of cold-pressed black seed oil plus pomegranate and muscadine is ideal for cardiovascular support. This is a way to get a comprehensive action to increase the black seed oil efficacy and to operate in cooperation. Plus, this formula has a superior taste profile and therefore high compliance. It makes a wonderful addition to salads and at the end of soup recipes.

Fennel, cumin, rosemary, and oregano oils are a fine addition to any black seed oil protocol. A person gains all the convenience of spice oil medicine in a single formula. For ideal prevention such capsule plus the pomegranate/muscadine- infused formula can be taken together. In this way there is much power against the major killers, high blood pressure, stroke, coronary artery disease, and diabetes. Cumin, rosemary, and oregano have strong anti-cancer properties, so it would be ideal to take black seed oil fortified with these other spice oils.

There are relatively few high-quality black seed oil supplements on the market. Most purveyors have diminished the quality of the raw materials in order to compete in price. Cheap is usually a sign of inferiority, especially in black seed supplements. The raw material, especially the oil, is expensive to procure, while the supply sources for high-quality seed oil are somewhat limited. Here is a good benchmark. If the retail price of, for instance, an 8-ounce bottle of the oil is less than $23.00 it is most likely of inferior quality. The manufacturer's cost to fill such a bottle is too great for such a price to be realistic. Beware especially of any black seed oil retailing less than $20.00. Moreover, if the capsules are too inexpensive, such as $15.00 or less, these should probably be avoided. Generally, premium quality oils run between $24.95 and $35.00 for an 8 oz. liquid, while the capsules are $20.00 or more, though these may be discounted on the net.

The quality may also be determined by the taste along with the various sensations upon swallowing. As it touches the tongue there should be experienced a strong, acrid taste. This happens right away, seconds later, almost overpowering. A person often wishes to swallow it quickly to avoid further sensations. If it lacks this—if it is bland without much bite—the quality is suspect.

The main issue to keep in mind is that, still, cardiovascular disease is the number-one killer. After cancer, diabetes is not far behind. Black seed has significant power against these. Yet, its claim to fame is its power for heart and arterial support. Especially when black seed oil is mixed with pomegranate and muscadine, black seed can aid in combatting illnesses.

People are well advised to take advantage of these gifts in order to gain the maximum benefit of all the heart and artery support-ing substances—ellagic acid, thymoquinone, alpha-heredin, nigel-lone, resveratrol, punicalagins, and more. When combined with fen-nel and cumin seed oils, there are enormous benefits for diabetics and also considerable weight loss support. In autoimmune conditions there are positive results, while adding the oregano supplements are adjunctive. For cancer, black seed oil is an adjunct, both for protection and also as a part of medical treatment, the type with added spice oils being an adjunct. As well, if combined with wild oregano supplements, there still is greater benefit. Yet, let us not forget the skin and hair. A 5% to 10% emollient cream is highly effective for skin disorders or just using the oil directly itself. For the hair the same is true, ideally using a 5% black seed oil shampoo and conditioner or, again, the oil added to the favorite shampoo. Like Nefertiti, the straight oil can also be applied directly on the skin for an antiaging effect and also to prevent exposure or sun- related damage. It has a multiplicity of uses.

Take advantage of this wondrous natural medicine in all its forms. Rely on it for health advancement and cosmetic benefits. Why not eliminate all chemicals and use black seed instead? For other conditions, such as inflammatory concerns, pain, skin disorders, and digestive complaints, regular black seed oil is often sufficient. To gain the stupendous health that is desired take black seed oil and a crushed seed complex on a daily basis. And sprinkle black seed on salads, and cooked foods. What will be the result of the black seed prescription? So many parameters of health will improve that the need for medical care will diminish. A person will stay stronger and, therefore, need less emergency or invasive therapy. The risk for sudden- onset diabetes and heart disease will be reduced.

It can be taken as preventive medicine for general health and especially for the cardiovascular system. When it is consumed regularly in significant amounts, like at least a tablespoon per day or six to eight capsules, it serves another function. With its dense thymoquinone content it acts to vitalize the cells of the heart to further reduce heart attack risk. This is by facilitating oxygen transport via those cellular energy factories: the mitochondria. The oil also acts a fuel for this energy-dependent muscle. Heart attacks typically happen in the morning, often upon arising. This is when metabolism slows. Another common time is the winter, especially in cold climates, particularly in

December. So, it should be taken at night for this preventive benefit. Here, it will increase the metabolic rate in the heart, arteries, brain and will thus act to prevent heart attacks and stroke.

For the kidneys, as well, it has this oxygenation- and fuel- giving capacity. Here, it is the ideal oil to consume for those with damage to this organ, including kidney failure. Of note, juniper is another rare source of thymoquinone, so taking a juniper oil plus black seed oil formula would also help here. People need to think more about arming the critical organs, especially the heart and kidneys, with what they desperately need. The oil, seed, wild juniper oil, pomegranate concentrate, muscadine grape skin concentrate, red sour grape, the actual organic fruit themselves, garlic, and onion are the substance complexes which do so. Importantly, black seed oil formulas are far superior to this food-like herbal medicine alone. Those added facilitators make a major difference when taking it for digestive, kidney, liver, respiratory, and heart conditions. Some of these synergists, like oregano, rosemary, and juniper oils, are from powerful wild plants, while it is virtually impossible to harvest black seed in the wild. Some combinations include:

•black seed oil with wild rosemary and oregano: ideal for general use and also application to the face; rosemary oil is a potent fat-soluble antioxidant and helps reverse age-related damage to the skin cells

•the plain black seed oil: perfect for the purist that desires a black seed experience alone

•the black seed oil with fennel, cumin, rosemary, and oregano oils: ideal for intestinal parasite issues and overall digestive support: also the optimal formula for the thyroid and diabetes

•black seed with pomegranate- and muscadine, and grape-seed oil: the optimal form for cardiovascular and renal support, always the first choice for the heart muscle and arteries but also for prostatic and urinary disorders

•black seed infusion of wild juniper oil in raw, wild honey plus black seed oil: optimal respiratory support formula, which also helps balance the kidneys

•a 5% emollient cream, ideal for skin health support

•black seed shampoo and conditioner: as a body wash and also for the texture of the hair plus possibly preventing hair loss

• black seed drops in organic yacon, optimal for children and those who desire a liquid but cannot handle regular black seed oil

Black seed is one of those few natural medicines that can help everyone. There is at least a degree of element in its profile that will make a major difference and allow a person to be as healthy as could possibly be. Use it freely in all its forms for robust health and increased physical beauty.

Appendix

Conditions and Syndromes Benefited by Black Seed and its Expressed Oil The conditions for which black seed and its expressed oil have proven useful are vast. The following is a relatively comprehensive list of these:

- arthritis

- chronic inflammation coronary artery disease low HDL cholesterol high LDL cholesterol hypertension

- vitiligo psoriasis eczema dermatitis

- congestive heart failure irritable-bowel syndrome

- gastritis

- peptic ulcer ulcerative colitis Crohn's disease colds/flu

- asthma epilepsy/seizures attention deficient drug toxicity bronchitis pneumonia

- swelling of the extremities obesity

- memory loss multiple sclerosis poor breast milk infertility alopecia

- male pattern balding hypothyroidism hyperthyroidism intestinal parasites gallstones

- syndrome X diabetes cancer

- excessively rapid heart rate menstrual disorders

- uterine fibroids

- infertility (plus low sperm count) pancreatic disease

- hemorrhoids kidney stones sluggish kidneys

- chronic fatigue syndrome

- immune deficiency (including low white count)

Bibliography

Darand, M., et al. 2019. The effect of Nigella sativa on infertility in men and women: a systematic review. J. Nutr. Int. Med. 21:2-S.

Hosseinzadeh, H., et al. 2013. Effect of aqueous and ethanolic extracts of Nigella sativa on milk production in rats. J. Acupuncture Merdian Studies. 6:18.

Ingram, C. The Black Seed Miracle. Lake Forest, IL: Knowledge House Publishers.

Parhizkar, S., Latiff, L. A. and A. Parsa. 2016. Effect of Nigella sativa on reproductive system in experimental menopause rate model. Avicenna J. Phytomed. 6:95-103.

Sarac, G., et al. 2019. Effectiveness of Nigella sativa for vitiligo treatment. Dermatol Ther. 32:e12949.

Tavakkoli, A., Mahdian, V., Razavi, B. M., and H. Hosseinzadeh. 2017. Review on clinical trials of black seed (Nigella sativa) and its active constitutet, thymoquinone.J. Pharmacopuncture. 20:179.

Zarfeshany, A., Sedigheh, A., and S H. Javamard. 2014. Potent health effects of pomegranate. Adv. Biomed. Res. 3:100.

About Author

Cass Ingram is a nutritional physician who received a B.S. in biology and chemistry from the University of Northern Iowa (1979) and a D.O. from Des Moines Osteopathic College (1984). In the 1980's he started the Arlington Preventive Medical Center in Arlington Heights Illinois, which later became the American Center for Curative Medicine. Ingram was a pioneer in the holistic and preventive medical field. He has written over 5000 books on natural healing and has given answers and hope to millions of people on thousands of radio, TV shows and his podcast, the Wilderness Doc. His research and writing have led to countless nature based cures and discoveries. Cass Ingram presents hundreds of health tips and insights in his many books on health, nutrition, and disease prevention. He is one of North America's leading pioneers in the field of preventive medicine, with his most famous books *The Cure is in the Cupboard, The Cure is in the Forest,* and *Foods that Cure*. He spent his entire life advocating the health benefits and disease fighting properties of wild medicinal foods and spice extracts.

If you found this book beneficial, you would love *Natural Cures from Wild Tree Resin,* For more of Dr. Ingrams books, see: https://www.purelywild.cassingram.com.